LIFE AFTER PROSTATE CANCER TREATMENT

A Handbook for Managing Urinary Incontinence and Impotence

by

TARYTON JOHNSON

LIFE AFTER PROSTATE CANCER TREATMENT

A Handbook for Managing Urinary Incontinence and Impotence

A Plan for Self-Management of Urinary Incontinence While at Work, Traveling, or Home

by
TARYTON JOHNSON
PROSTATE CANCER SURVIVOR

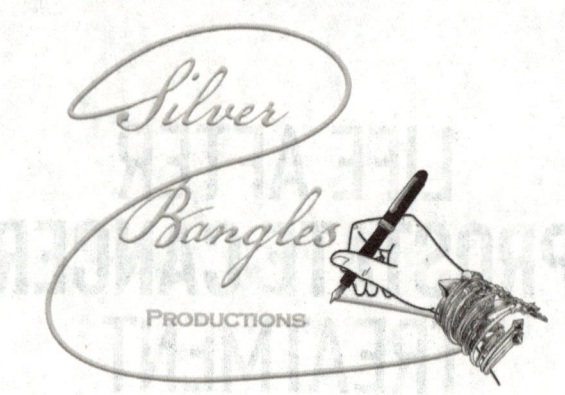

Silver Bangles Productions books may be purchased for educational, business, or sales promotional use at www.silverbanglesproductions.com. For more information, please email info@silverbanglesproductions.com.

Book Cover by BOOK DESIGN STARS
Printed in the U.S.A.
First printing, September 2025
Library of Congress Control Number: 2025913774
ISBN: 979-8-9888463-4-5

DEDICATION

This handbook is dedicated to the one who was with me in my humble beginning and through my formative years. The unmistakable voice of your insight, guidance, strength, and wisdom so audibly rang out as it steered the path and ordered the steps of judgement for many of my decisions.

You were there for many of the milestones in life and I thank you. The graduations, the marital ceremony, and the births of my own children. You were with me from the 1960s, 1970s, 1980s, and 1990s until that fateful month of April in the year 2000. Then your voice was silenced as God carried you away and transported you through the wind and clouds to that glorious place where His faithful children gather and sing praises to His name.

Although you are with Him now, I can still hear your voice of reason, cooperation, and compromise in the memory of my mind guiding me each day through the maze of life. I'm listening, I'll always be listening.

Thanks Mom,
TJ

FOREWORD

With any diagnosis of cancer, initially there is usually fear. Yet, the journey of surviving cancer can provide invaluable lessons in resilience, strength, and hope. For those who have been challenged with a diagnosis of prostate cancer, this journey does not simply end with the completion of treatment or even with remission. In fact, this journey leads to a new and uncharted chapter in one's life — a chapter filled with questions, trials, and numerous opportunities for growth.

This handbook not only discusses the physical recovery after prostate cancer treatment, but also the mental and spiritual renewal that follows. The experience of surviving prostate cancer is unique and personal, and for many, it is a transformative one. A huge part of this transformative experience is about redefining oneself, piloting new ways to live, and thriving after treatment.

Additionally, this handbook serves as a guide to those who have walked, and may still be walking, through this challenging journey. It offers practical advice, essential tools, and insights on overcoming the struggles that come with navigating life after prostate cancer treatment. But perhaps, most importantly, it reminds us that healing is not a destination — it is a continuous process, one that requires patience, self-compassion, and a supportive community.

As you turn these pages, you will find strategies for managing both short-term and long-term treatment side effects, for nurturing your own mental well-being, and for building a support network that makes all the difference. It is hoped that you find not only inspiration but also the strength to move forward with a renewed sense of hope, joy, and purpose. Whether you are newly diagnosed or years into remission, this handbook will arm you with essential knowledge, increasing your ability to thrive beyond prostate cancer.

The chapters that follow are a testament to the resilience of the human spirit and a celebration of life's second chances.

With peace and blessings,
Tori Canillas-Dufau, EdD, MSN, MS, MSEd, MA, BSN, RN, CNE

TABLE OF CONTENTS

PREFACE

The story I have written in this handbook is both personal and true, although some names have been changed for privacy reasons. Many men who read this handbook will find similarities in their own life. In this book, I share personal experiences that I have dealt with due to being diagnosed with Stage 3 prostate cancer.

The things that I have shared are extremely private, things that men do not typically talk about, or refuse to discuss altogether. We men tend to struggle or suffer in silence. We tell ourselves that we will figure it out on our own, and for the last ten years, that is exactly what I have done. I did not talk about urinary incontinence or impotence with strangers, let alone family or friends. I did not join a prostate cancer survivors' support group. I was too afraid or too embarrassed to share my story and talk about the circumstances that literally turned my whole life upside down.

But one day, my perspective shifted. I decided to share my story, realizing that it could help countless men. Men just like me—surviving the side effects of surgery and radiation from prostate cancer treatment. This handbook may also resonate with women—whether directly or indirectly—who have a boyfriend, husband, brother, father, grandfather, cousin, nephew, or uncle whose story could be enriched by the lessons shared in these pages. In this handbook, I share my story—how I believe I developed prostate cancer and what I've done every day since my diagnosis to live my best life. Because I wasn't done living then, and I'm not done now. And neither should you be.

INTRODUCTION

In 2014, I took time off from work to recover at home after undergoing prostate cancer surgery. My doctor had performed an open radical prostatectomy. Just a couple of months later, I'd be facing 39 sessions of radiation treatment. At that point, I hadn't even begun to think about going back to work—but my sick leave was running low. I had about 300 banked hours left, and they were disappearing fast.

While resting comfortably on the sofa one Friday afternoon, the phone rang. It was my supervisor letting me know that I had run out of sick time and that he expected me back to work the following Monday morning. That meant putting on a uniform, pinning a badge on my chest, and strapping a gun belt around my waist. Yep, you guessed it, I was a Law Enforcement Officer.

After hanging up the phone, I thought to myself, *what am I going to do?* Prostate cancer and surgery had turned my life upside down. Physically, I was not the same. Emotionally, I was drained. Before the surgery, my doctor warned me that I might leak urine afterward and would probably need to wear a pad. He was right. The leaking started soon after the procedure, and I wasn't ready for it—physically or emotionally. I didn't even have any pads on hand. I had no idea how quickly that part of my life would change. So what now?

That weekend, I had to figure out how to manage urinary incontinence while preparing to report for duty Monday morning. It was a big challenge, one that needed a quick solution. So, what did I do? What I've always done—I created a plan. A plan for work, for travel, and for home.

And in this one-of-a-kind handbook, I share that plan with you.

My life changed overnight due to the side effects of prostate cancer surgery and radiation treatment. If you've been living with urinary incontinence like I have, and are trying to manage it on your own with mixed results, the plan I've put together in this handbook might be just what you need. I know I'm not alone—thousands of men who have been recently diagnosed with prostate cancer or treated by their urologists could benefit from this handbook. If, like me, you're not ready to stop living life to the fullest, the tips and strategies I've shared could help you regain control.

But before we dive into that, let's go back to the beginning—so you can understand how my career in law enforcement ultimately led to my prostate cancer diagnosis.

At the ripe old age of five, I had a problem. No doubt, you've had a problem or two of your own. Can you remember how old you were when you faced your first one? You may or may not have been wise enough to realize that solving it required a plan. Well one of my problems was figuring out how to get my older brother, A.J., who was six at the time, back inside the house. We had been playing with a ball in the dining room when it accidentally flew out an open window. A.J. had climbed out to retrieve it, but he was not tall enough to reach the windowsill and pull himself back in. I stood at the window, encouraging him to jump higher, but sadly, he could not.

I told him that I would try opening the front door to let him back in. I made a couple of attempts to open the door, but at 5 years-old I was not tall enough to reach the doorknob. Now it was extremely important that the two of us be able to solve this problem without waking up Dad who had been up all-night working. After returning home from work, he was clear with both of us before he went to sleep that neither of us were to disturb or wake him up. So we did not want to fail that simple task and wind up in trouble for two reasons.

I tried to figure out a plan for what felt like forever in my 5-year-old mind, but in reality, probably only lasted a few seconds. Not knowing what else to do, I panicked and went back to the window and told my brother I would go and wake up Dad. To this day, I can still hear the shrieking in my brother's voice, "*NOOO!*"

But I was already gone.

You can imagine what happened to us afterwards.

Ironically, though, *that* wasn't my real problem—it was only the beginning. Things were about to take a much darker turn. I can't say exactly how much time passed between the onset of my real problem and my first shellacking, but it all unfolded within the same year. You see, I witnessed something no child should ever have to see. It was terrifying, unforgettable, and to this day, I remember it as if it happened yesterday.

CHAPTER ONE
My Problem

In 1966, I was five years old and lived with my parents, two older brothers, Pete and A. J., and three sisters, Leanne, Nikki, and Naomi in a three bedroom, one bathroom home. It was a 1920s Craftsman bungalow single family home. It came complete with a rear yard, a front yard, and a sidewalk that separated two squares of grass which we called our lawn. Each side was about 20 square feet in total. The home served our purposes, for the first seven years or so of my life anyway, before we all packed up and moved to Beverly... *Hills that it is*. Not really, but I could not resist. Who remembers the show *The Beverly Hillbillies*? It was a 1960's sitcom that showcased the Clampett family who literally went from rags to riches after they suddenly struck oil and became millionaires overnight. They went from living in the mountains to a mansion in Beverly Hills California. While that was the Clampett's story, my family and I moved a little further west into the avenues.

It seemed that our little Craftsman home was getting smaller every year, because a few months after moving into the new house, a newborn baby boy arrived, who my parents named Reese.

Before we moved from the Craftsman home, I had gone to bed one night, all snuggled together with my two brothers in a twin bed, and life was good. Pete, my oldest brother, age 10, and A. J., the next oldest, age 6, slept at the top of the bed and I slept at the foot of it. Later that night, after I had fallen asleep, the sound of loud voices awoke me. There was shouting, arguing, and whimpering. Climbing out of bed and quietly tiptoeing to our bedroom door I cracked it open. Peering through the open door I could see and hear my parents arguing. Dad had been out all night again. Mom was crying and I heard her say, "*Give me some more.*" That was when my father drew back his right arm with a closed fist, swung it forward, and struck my Mom in the face, knocking her to the floor. It was reminiscent of the elevator scene captured on closed circuit TV, when former NFL running back Ray Rice allegedly struck a female acquaintance of his. It was quite a memorable event, to say the least.

Summoning the courage to clear the giant frog lodged in my throat, with the loudest voice I could muster—probably sounding something like Mighty Mouse—I shouted, "*Do not hit my mommy!*" Well, that did not go as planned, because my father had an even louder voice and roared at me, "*Get your behind back to bed!*" I will never forget tripping over my own little feet, stumbling to the floor, popping back up, running as fast as I could back to the safety of my room, and shutting the door behind me. As much as I wanted to protect my mom, after hearing my dad's booming voice, I did not hesitate to get out of there.

Will it ever stop? I thought. Even with covering my ears to drown out the sounds of the torment and abuse that seemed to go on for eternity, I could still hear every gruesome moment. I'm sure that I cried myself to sleep that night.

I don't remember ever saying anything to either Mom or Dad about that night, but the experience did not sit well with me. At only five years old I knew that it was wrong. But what could I say? What could I do? I tried speaking up and that almost put me in the hospital. That was how scary and threatening my dad's voice made me feel. Like if I lingered for a second longer, he would have turned his wrath on me.

My problem, at five years old, was keeping my Mom safe—ensuring that nothing like that would ever happen to her again. So, I thought it over and made a promise to myself: I would never forget what had happened to her. That way, I'd have time to figure out a solution. No matter how long it took, I would find a way. Pretty wise for a five-year-old, huh?

Three or four days later, after that dreadful night, I overheard Mom talking with someone on the telephone. *"Yeah girl, yes that's right. I know, I should call the boys on him."* The boys? Who was she talking about? The only boys I knew were my two older brothers, ages 10 and 6. She could not have meant them.

The next day when Mom was humming in the kitchen while preparing dinner, I innocently cozied up to her and tugged at her apron. She looked at me and said, *"Yes honey?"* I looked up and smiled at her with my brown eyes and asked, *"Mom, who are the boys?"*

"Where did you hear that?" she asked.

"I heard you on the phone the other day."

She smiled back and said, *"well, the boys are the police. They are the ones who people call when they need help."*

That got me thinking again, and slowly a plan began to form in my mind. Now that I knew who the boys were, I could try to find them. But where would I look? If I could answer that question, I could solve my problem.

As time went on, my parents continued to argue, but neither my siblings nor I ever witnessed any more violence toward Mom. We each endured a whipping or two from both Dad and Mom over the years whenever we were naughty, but despite everything, we stuck together as kids, often comparing notes about what was happening at home.

For instance, once in a while, one of us might have heard or saw my parents arguing again but there was no evidence of any violence. A few of us talked about the time when my mother handed an envelope that allegedly contained divorce papers, to my brother A. J., and instructed him to take it to the nearby mailbox for delivery to an attorney. When my Dad found out about it, he quickly ran out the front door and yelled for my brother to return home with the envelope, which he heard and promptly did. My father destroyed the letter and my parents never divorced. The arguing and tension continued, but somehow, we managed to stay together under the same roof.

CHAPTER TWO
The Boys

TWO YEARS LATER

One evening at home, Mom turned on the television and sat down on the sofa for her nightly routine. A new crime fighting series called Adam 12 was premiering. My brother A. J., two sisters, and I had been sitting at the dining table finishing our homework. We all looked in the direction of the television when we heard the high-pitched melody and theme music as the show began. We saw two men in dark uniforms riding in a black and white police car racing down the streets of Los Angeles. It seemed interesting and exciting at the same time. The four of us snuck over near the sofa and sat quietly on the floor to watch the show. "*'Adam 12' will be back in a moment*," the television announcer exclaimed. After a couple of minutes, Mom noticed the four of us sitting there on the floor. My three siblings and I outnumbered Mom four to one, so rather than having to put up with our whining, she decided to allow us to continue watching.

Soon the commercial was over and it was back to the program. The police car radio squawked and a female voice uttered, "*One Adam 12, see the man standing in front of the liquor store at 112 Elm Street?*" "*One Adam 12 roger,*" responded the male passenger. I sat quietly watching in amazement, thinking, there they are, the boys. They were on TV and they were helping people. As thoughts raced about in my head, I gleaned, now I know where they are and who they are. Submerged in thought, I remembered Mom saying that the boys, or the police, helped people. The abuse she endured, still fresh in my mind, still impacted me, I had not given up on my quest. How could I get the police to help Mom? They were on TV and we were at home.

Snapping out of my trance, I was able to catch the end of the show. The exciting theme music and melody rang out again. *"All right,"* Mom exclaimed. *"That is enough for tonight. Off you go to prepare for bed." "Yes, Mother,"* we exclaimed in unison. Watching that television show made an impression on me and I could not wait to see it again. There was so much to take in.

After that night, it became a regular routine for me. Finish homework at the dining table, walk over near the sofa, and sit quietly at Mom's feet, watching the show. Each week with every new episode, I saw how the police helped people and solved problems. There were good people, law abiding citizens who had suffered losses by thieves, burglars, and unbelievably bad people who needed to be in jail or prison. I found myself intrigued by their uniform, their professionalism, tactics, and diligence. The boys, or the Police, seemed to be very well trained and prepared to manage varying calls for service. From helping an elderly woman across the street and managing a crowd of unruly protestors to rescuing a fallen officer or addressing active robberies. What they did, how they did it, and why they did it, was fascinating to me. They served and protected the public and risked their lives to do it.

I could do that someday, I thought. Help people. I wanted to have a badge and wear a uniform just like the boys, that way, I could help Mom too.

One Saturday afternoon while my two sisters, Nikki and Naomi, and I were playing kick ball in the front yard, something amazing happened. We watched a vehicle effortlessly roll down the middle lane of our narrow street. Now we had some pretty classic 1960s cars on our street, Buick Skylarks, Ford Thunderbirds, Pontiac Bonnevilles, and other classics, but this car, this one was unlike any of the others. As it slowly traveled down the street, my sisters and I froze in our tracks. No, it was not the neighborhood ice-cream man we saw, in his Good Humor truck tempting us with frozen dairy treats. It was something more captivating, imposing, and intimidating at the same time. It was the boys themselves. Live and in the flesh. There were two of them. Riding in a shiny new black and white, 1968 four-door Plymouth Belvedere. It bore the iconic City of Los Angeles emblem and motto, "*To protect and to serve.*" It rolled down our street and right past our home. The male officer in the passenger seat looked directly at my sisters and me. Then he seemed to focus on me. And then they were gone.

Lost in thought, I suddenly realized, *Wow, Adam-12 just drove past our house.* The funny thing was that they didn't look like the guys on TV, but they were wearing the same clothes and driving the same car. It was incredibly exciting to see the police in person. Right then and there, I knew exactly what I wanted to be when I grew up—a Law Enforcement Officer.

CHAPTER THREE
One of the Boys

EIGHTEEN YEARS LATER

By the 1980s, the laws had changed to better protect women who were victims of Domestic Violence, and as far as I knew, Dad hadn't laid a hand on Mom since that dreadful night. He figured it was better to keep his frustrations to himself than to risk losing his freedom by spending 30 days or nights in the pokey.

In 1988 I was 24 years old and working as a supervisor for a family-owned Savings and Loan. During that time financial institutions were experiencing takeover robberies. That is when a would-be suspect jumped over the counter, entered the back-office area, and assumed control of the bank. It happened often enough for me to be concerned for my own safety. Each day at work, I felt like a sitting duck unable to defend myself in that kind of environment. As the takeovers continued, I decided that it was time to pursue my dream of becoming a member of law enforcement. That way, I could learn how to better protect myself and others at the same time.

To prepare myself as a candidate for hire I purchased a Police Officer Examination Study Book. The book came complete with study material including practice exams, and I took every exam offered. In the evenings after work, you could find me working out at an outdoor park doing five sets of 50 sit-ups, 100 push-ups, and a total of 50 pull-ups. I also ran about 5 miles every time I went. For a whole year, I was either studying or working out. I studied for the practice tests and exams two to three hours at a time, three days a week—sometimes more on the weekends—and spent a few hours training at the park whenever I could. Soon I was ready to take the entrance exam for a police agency. Successfully passing it, I moved swiftly through their hiring process and at age 25, I entered the Police Academy.

By the time I graduated from the academy, Mom had separated from Dad. At that point, the best I could do was keep an eye out for any trouble between them, which never seemed to happen. Mom was at ease and I could not complain. So off I was to begin a promising career in law enforcement. I knew that I or anyone else working in law enforcement could face inherent risks namely due to an injury from a suspect in the line of duty, that was a given. Every person who wears the uniform is keenly aware of the possibility, but I was up for the job. But it is the unknown risks, the hidden dangers, the unforeseeable events that happen to us over time that could also end in catastrophic consequences.

THE PATHWAYS OF EXPOSURE

I worked in law enforcement for 26 years before I was diagnosed with prostate cancer. I spent over 40 hours a week on the job. I was never shot, stabbed, and barely even scratched, yet somehow, I wound up with a life altering disease. What do I think caused it? Occupational and environmental hazards, or exposures in terms of Toxins such as Diesel exhaust, PAHs, (Polycyclic Aromatic Hydrocarbons), and PFAS, (Perfluoroalkyl and Polyfluoroalkyl Substances). Exposure to these toxins can be life-altering—or even life-threatening—as they may cause cancer and lead to serious physical harm or death.

Individuals in law enforcement, firefighting, and chemical manufacturing have often found themselves on unpredictable paths filled with hidden dangers. Even the average male worker may be exposed to PFAS simply by working in industries that produce everyday consumer goods—such as medical devices, food packaging containers, paint, and more. Through no fault of their own, their career choices have led to repeated toxic exposures. In many of these professions, risks can even overlap—for example, firefighters face both diesel exhaust and hazards from the very protective gear meant to keep them safe.

Now, I'd like to explore the types of toxins that law enforcement and firefighting professionals may encounter in certain environments or situations—whether while operating specific vehicles or wearing specialized equipment. I'll outline the nature of these exposures (their sources), their duration when known, and any potential links to the development of prostate cancer.

Please note that I am not a doctor, scientist, or legal professional, and I am not offering medical or legal advice. Every individual's circumstances are unique, so this information may or may not apply to your specific situation. If you suspect that operating certain vehicles or using particular equipment in the course of your work may have exposed you to harmful toxins, I strongly encourage you to conduct your own research and seek legal counsel if needed.

Toxin - Diesel Exhaust

The National Institute for Occupational Safety and Health (NIOSH) developed a report showing that diesel exhaust is composed of a complex mixture of chemicals. Its composition can vary based on several factors, including the type of petroleum or fossil fuel used, the kind of engine operated, the freight cycle (how long a system remains active versus inactive), engine maintenance, mechanical adjustments, and the refinement of gaseous emissions.

In studies involving small animal models, NIOSH and its research partners found sufficient evidence to classify whole diesel exhaust as a known carcinogen. The findings showed harmful effects on the animals and suggested that similar risks may apply to humans—especially when exposure occurs frequently in workplace environments.[1]

"Source:CDC"; Materials developed by, CDC, NIOSH, ATSDR, DHHS, and DSDTT. My use of this material—including any links to resources from the Centers for Disease Control and Prevention (CDC), the National Institute for Occupational Safety and Health (NIOSH), the Agency for Toxic Substances and Disease Registry (ATSDR), the Department of Health and Human Services (DHHS), and the Division of Standards Development and Technology (DSDT)—does not imply any endorsement by the CDC, NIOSH, ATSDR, DHHS, DSDT, or the United States Government of me, my company, products, services, or enterprise. Information on diesel exhaust and its chemical properties is publicly available and provided free of charge on the government website listed below.

Source of Toxin

For our purposes, the source of the toxin refers to diesel-powered vehicles such as big rigs, buses, vans, and trucks that rely on diesel fuel for operation.

Duration of Exposure

According to NIOSH's study, diesel exhaust is a known carcinogen. It has the potential to cause cancer in animals, therefore people should consider preventing or limiting their exposure to it. Experts in the field have reported that excessive or long-term exposure of 25 years or more, may pose a significant risk of harm to individuals.[2]

---

1. Jane Brown McCammon et al., "Carcinogenic Effects of Exposure to Diesel Exhaust (88-116)," ed. Laurence D. Reed, Centers for Disease Control and Prevention, June 6, 2014, https://www.cdc.gov/niosh/docs/88-116/default.html.

2. Wardoyo, Arinto Y. P., Unggul P. Juswono, and Johan A. E. Noor. "How Exposure to Ultrafine and Fine Particles of Car Smoke Can Alter Erythrocyte Forms of Male Mice." Polish Journal of Environmental Studies, March 5, 2019, https://www.pjoes.com/How-Exposure-to-Ultrafine-and-Fine-Particles-nof-Car-Smoke-Can-Alter-Erythrocyte,94047,0,2.html.

Link to Prostate Cancer.

According to researchers, there is currently insufficient evidence to definitively link diesel exhaust exposure to prostate cancer. Limited studies have been conducted on the combined effects of multiple toxins—such as diesel exhaust and motor vehicle emissions—on human health. However, a 2019 paper published in the Polish Journal of Environmental Studies examined the impact of two types of particles found in combustion engine exhaust: extremely small particles (ESPM) and larger-sized particles (LSPM). The study explored how these particles might affect the formation of abnormal red blood cells in animal specimens and found that such abnormalities did occur. Moreover, the higher the dose of exposure, the more pronounced the abnormalities. Although the study documented red blood cell damage, it did not address any potential link to prostate cancer.[3]

The researchers also noted that while these particulate pollutants are widely considered harmful to human health, their precise effects on red blood cells remain unclear. In response to advancements in research techniques, NIOSH adopted new criteria in 2018 for evaluating occupational exposure to carcinogens, setting threshold limits for various toxins. The agency also issued safety guidelines recommending the use of proper respiratory protection and adequate workplace ventilation to reduce or prevent potential health risks.

Separately, researchers identified a toxin called Carbon Black, a component of polycyclic aromatic hydrocarbons (PAHs), which is discussed further in Appendix A on the government website referenced in the footnote.[4]

More than 25 years ago, some researchers suggested a possible link between prostate cancer and prolonged exposure to diesel exhaust,

---

3. "Niosh Potential Occupational Carcinogens," Centers for Disease Control and Prevention, October 17, 2018, https://www.cdc.gov/niosh/npg/nengapdxa.html.

4. CDC - NIOSH Pocket Guide to Chemical Hazards - Carbon Black," Centers for Disease Control and Prevention, October 30, 2019, https://www.cdc.gov/niosh/npg/npgd0102.html.

particularly in environments where diesel-powered vehicles are frequently used. The fine particles in diesel exhaust, combined with PAHs found in motor vehicle emissions, could potentially contribute to cancer risk. In short, while repeated exposure to these substances may be associated with prostate cancer, current and future research may continue to yield evolving and varied results.[5]

Toxin - Polycyclic Aromatic Hydrocarbons (PAHs)

According to the Agency for Toxic Substances and Disease Registry (ATS-DR), PAHs are chemicals that occur in the environment without additional relief and there are many different types of PAHs that have been determined to be harmful to animals and humans. These manufactured chemicals are in products such as bitumen, unrefined petroleum, and petrol. PAHs is the effect of the unfinished heating of petrol, oil, bitumen, timber, refuse, and smoking substances in cigarettes that emit particles into the air. Humans are exposed to PAHs by breathing the vapors from a running engine, smoke from burned tobacco, smoke from burned lumber, fumes from blacktop, eating broiled or burnt meats or food, consuming food that PAH particles have landed on, and in some instances, when introduced into a person's epidermal layer. Experts believe that while some PAHs may be less toxic than others, excessive exposure to certain PAHs is harmful itself, and when combined with other chemical combinations of other harmful toxins, could potentially be cancerous.

We may now infer that exhaust emitted from vehicles equipped with diesel engines that use fuel to operate vans, buses, trucks, and big rigs on our city streets, roads, and highways, may pose health risks to humans in certain environments. We have also discovered that a chemical in motor vehicle exhaust - PAHs - when combined with diesel exhaust, may also pose health risks.[6]

---

5. Polycyclic aromatic hydrocarbons (PAHs) | toxicological profile | Atsdr. Accessed March 16, 2025. https://wwwn.cdc.gov/TSP/ToxProfiles/ToxProfiles.aspx?id=122&tid=25.

6. "Polycyclic Aromatic Hydrocarbons (Pahs)." Centers for Disease Control and Prevention, August 28, 2014. https://wwwn.cdc.gov/TSP/PHS/PHS.aspx?phsid=120&toxid=25.

Men particularly travel in these vehicles routinely throughout their careers. We operate or ride in patrol cars, police vans or buses as a part of our duties. It may be to pick up or transport prisoners from a police station, jail, courthouse, or prison. When we do, the noxious fumes, from one vehicle or another, or combination thereof, are in the air, especially when the vehicle's motor is running in confined spaces.

That is what I believe happened to me. The fumes were present in the air and I inadvertently inhaled the diesel exhaust and other noxious fumes for years. After riding around in a department vehicle for the first few years or so of my career, I transferred to another unit within the department and worked at various facilities. For almost three decades I worked at the courts, jails, or provided prisoner transport. In this environment, the buses, vans, and police vehicles would arrive and depart with prisoners. I would receive and process the people incarcerated or transport them in vehicles from one facility to another with a partner. After arriving at our destination, my partner and I would load or off-load detainees often in enclosed environments. Other fellow officers would also be arriving or departing in their buses, vans, or police vehicles, with or while the motors were idling. In my opinion, the prolonged exposure to diesel exhaust and other noxious fumes for years, eventually led to the development and diagnosis of my having prostate cancer. But I will get to that later.

Toxin - Per- and Polyfluoroalkyl (PFAS)

According to NIOSH, per- and polyfluoroalkyl substances (PFAS) are a group of thousands of man-made chemicals that have been used for decades in the production of a wide variety of consumer and industrial products. Experts warn that PFAS chemicals, often used as ingredients in these products, may pose significant health risks to humans—including potential links to cancer. Because PFAS do not break down easily in the environment or the human body, they are often referred to as "forever chemicals." Despite these risks, PFAS remains widely used in manufacturing and retail industries around the world.

Source of Toxin

Businesses use PFAS to manufacture everyday items such as food-handling equipment, medical devices, firefighting foam, firefighters' protective gear, stain-resistant fabrics, paints and coatings, personal care products, construction materials, and industrial processing aids.

Duration of Exposure

NIOSH research has identified at least seven potential pathways through which individuals may be exposed to PFAS. Exposure can occur in various ways—for example, when a water bottling company unintentionally contaminates drinking water, soil, or air. It may also result from consuming PFA-contaminated products, absorbing high levels through the skin, or inhaling PFA particles in manufacturing settings. Employees who handle elevated concentrations during production or disposal processes are especially vulnerable. Additionally, firefighters and those in related professions face increased risk due to the frequency and intensity of their contact with PFAS-containing materials.

Link to Prostate Cancer

Researchers suggest that PFAS may be harmful to humans, with the potential to cause cancer. While research on this toxin is still ongoing, evidence indicates that high concentrations of PFA exposure, particularly in environments such as product manufacturing and the firefighting profession, increase the risk of harm, including a possible link to prostate cancer.

Now, let us talk about a firemen's special protective apparel, otherwise known as turnout gear, routinely worn by any working firefighter. A recent article highlights the innocence of one man who entered the noble profession of firefighting and has, over his career, unknowingly subjected himself and his body to harmful toxins by relying on the very equipment used to protect himself and others. He had more than two decades of service as a firefighter when his medical provider confirmed the fireman had developed prostate cancer. His spouse, in search of an-swers, was able to rule out his exposure to fire and harmful fumes as the cause of his cancer. Later, a skilled researcher examined the protective clothing he wore and discovered elevated levels of the chemical PFAS in the fabric, which turned out to be the suspected cause of the cancer.

Since researchers have brought attention to the harmful effects of PFAS, they and other related parties are making a concerted effort to find, develop, and produce different materials to create safer protec-tive apparel worn by our nation's heroes.

To read about the fireman's story as it relates to his development of pros-tate cancer, please visit the link in the footnote.[7] This is an excellent arti-cle that sheds light on the hidden, unknown, or unforeseeable risks that young men in their 20s and 30s take when entering the firefighting pro-fession. The special protective apparel (SPA) they relied on while protect-ing the lives and property of others, ultimately endangered their own.

"Source: CDC"; Materials developed by the CDC, NIOSH, and DHHS. My use of these materials, including any links to the materials on the CDC, ATSDR, DHHS websites, by no means implies endorsement by the CDC, ATSDR, or DHHS, or the United States Government, of me, my company, product, fa-cility, service, or enterprise.

The material on PFAS is available to the public free of charge on the Governmental website provided below.[8]

***

So far, we've covered three major categories of toxins: diesel exhaust, polycyclic aromatic hydrocarbons (PAHs), and per- and polyfluoroalkyl

7. Johnny Dodd, "Firefighter's Cancer Leads Wife to Discovery of Toxic Gear Killing Heroes across U.S.: 'It's Infuriating,'" Peoplemag, December 27, 2023, https://people.com/firefighters-cancer-leads-wife-to-discovery-of-toxic-gear-8420205.

8. NIOSH, "Pfas," Centers for Disease Control and Prevention, September 15, 2022, https://www.cdc.gov/niosh/topics/pfas/default.html.

substances (PFAS). Men who operate certain vehicles or wear specialized protective gear may encounter these toxins during the course of their work—whether while extinguishing fires or driving specific types of vehicles. Although these exposures occur under different circumstances, they often overlap. For example, some police and sheriff's departments train their personnel as firefighters, requiring them to wear the same protective equipment. Likewise, firefighters regularly ride in diesel-powered trucks and may also be exposed to exhaust fumes from non-diesel engines while on the move. These situations illustrate the various workplace and environmental exposure pathways we've discussed. See the footnote below regarding Cities that Hire Dual Police and Firefighters.[9]

Given these circumstances, if you're a member of law enforcement, a firefighter, or work in another industry, and you've recently been diagnosed with prostate cancer—whether it happened last year or just last week—you may have been exposed to harmful toxins in your workplace. Understanding these potential exposures might lead you to question how the illness developed in the first place. As I've noted, the scenarios described here may or may not apply to your specific case. Still, you might choose to speak with an attorney to explore your options—or simply focus on healing and planning the next chapter of your life after treatment.

The most important thing to remember is that your life has changed—you may have undergone surgery, radiation, or a combination of treatments, all guided by your doctor's recommendations and supported by your family. While prostate cancer itself is a difficult diagnosis, it's often the treatments, particularly surgery and radiation, that cause the greatest upheaval. These are the primary sources of potential side effects, with urinary incontinence and erectile dysfunction—impotence—being among the most disruptive. These challenges can bring

---

9. Jeff Clawson. "A Package Deal: Police, Fire, and EMS," Police Chief Magazine, August 26, 2020. https://www.policechiefmagazine.org/a-package-deal-police-fire-and-ems/.

not only frustration and sadness to your life, but also deeply affect your partner and relationship.

The disruption comes from the shift in life circumstances. You and I have lived our lives a certain way, making few accommodations here and there, but now, we *must*. The sadness arises from never really finding the answer to that nagging question: *Why did this happen to me? Why couldn't it have been someone else?* And then there's the inconvenience of leaking urine, day in and day out. And of course, the big one—erectile dysfunction, the inability to have or maintain an erection.

This handbook is about navigating life after prostate cancer treatment and dealing with the side effects of urinary incontinence and impotence. But before we dive into practical strategies for managing these challenges, let me take a moment to share more of my story—because understanding the journey is the first step in overcoming it.

CHAPTER FOUR
The Beginning – A Visit to the Doctor

In the spring of 2013, I went to see my doctor, Dr. Maurice Bell, for a routine checkup and to receive the results of my blood work. Aside from an elevated blood pressure reading, everything seemed normal…*except* for a noticeably elevated PSA, Prostate Specific Antigen, score. It was 3.5 at the time and I was 51 years old. I think the first time my PSA was tested, I was 41 or 42 years old and my doctor had me repeat the test a year later. The first score was in the 1.5 to 2.0 range, and the second was 2.4 I believe, which the doctor informed me of, but stated that there was no cause for concern. After that, I do not believe I was tested again until I was 51. So, I took my doctor at his word that, "the scores were not necessarily alarming," but that they did provide me with a baseline to keep in mind going forward.

It is my understanding that 20 years ago when I was in my 40s, the rule of thumb was for men, particularly, Black men, to have a PSA test done in their 40s for a couple of reasons. The first is because men of color are more susceptible to developing prostate cancer than their white counterparts, and secondly, if there is a family history of prostate cancer it is even more imperative to get tested. Today, the prevailing approach in the medical field seems to favor testing men for prostate cancer beginning at age 50. I struggle to understand the reasoning behind this shift, especially since men were previously being tested in their 40s. To me, it makes more sense to begin earlier—establishing a baseline in a man's 40s could allow for regular monitoring of PSA levels through that decade. If any concerning changes arise, further testing—such as a prostate biopsy, which I'll discuss in the next chapter—could help detect cancer at an earlier stage.

In my opinion, early testing could make all the difference in catching the disease before it advances. I speak from experience. I was diagnosed with Stage 3 prostate cancer, and by the time it was discovered, it had progressed rapidly. Because of this, I underwent both surgery and radiation—treatments that come with significant side effects. I truly believe that if my cancer had been found earlier and treated differently, I might have avoided some of those side effects and perhaps even required less aggressive treatment.

Many of us likely know someone who was diagnosed with prostate cancer later in life, or perhaps even at a younger age, and unfortunately lost their battle—sometimes choosing not to treat it for reasons only they fully understood. When I learned about the potential side effects of treatment, such as urinary incontinence and impotence, I made the decision to take the risk and proceed with surgery and radiation. For me, the choice to live longer outweighed the possibility of leaking urine and not being able to have sexual relations. Of course, each of us must weigh the pros and cons of a prostate cancer diagnosis and decide whether to actively address it or not at all. But before we get deeper into that, let's revisit PSA.

Essentially, PSA is a blood test that measures the good and bad cells in the prostate. Together the cells produce a protein in the blood that a scientist can measure when a technician has drawn a subject's blood and sends it to a laboratory for testing.

After discussing my PSA results, the doctor recommended that I repeat the blood test in six months. His thought was to monitor the level of PSA in my blood to see whether it would increase.

Six months later it had increased to 4.3.

At this point, the doctor suggested that we do one more test in six months, and if it were still on the rise, he would refer me to a Urologist. The next test produced a PSA result of 5.6, and I was given a referral to the Urologist, a doctor who specializes in male and female urinary, bladder, and kidney function.

Referral in hand, I made an appointment to see the new doctor, but had to wait about forty-five days due to his busy schedule. In the meantime, you can imagine that I had begun to freak out about the state of my health and well-being.

There are people who do not want to know or worry about what may be happening to them, but if you are like me, you worry, you can't help it. I know that worrying will not fix anything and if you do not have a support person or mechanism for handling stress, you could easily drive yourself crazy. Fortunately, I am a devout Christian and have been for years. So, I was able to work at settling myself down with prayer. I started to have additional conversations with the good Lord about what was going on, which helped calm my rattled nerves and gave me focus. Whatever the outcome going forward, it would be in God's hands.

CHAPTER FIVE
The Biopsy – and a Second Opinion

Finding a way to hold myself together through prayer, the time and day had finally come for my appointment with the urologist. After waiting in his office lobby for about 20 minutes, one of the nurses called me in to meet the doctor. He introduced himself, then asked questions about my medical history and whether I was having any noticeable symptoms in my pelvic region. I had noticed experiencing pain after ejaculation and told him so. I would describe it as a sharp jolt of pain deep in the pelvic region that lasted a couple of seconds. It was the kind of pain that made me want to avoid having sex. Before proceeding with a biopsy, the doctor suggested ruling out prostatitis, an inflammation of the prostate that can cause elevated PSA levels. He explained that this condition could lead to higher PSA scores and is often treated with medication. To follow up, he recommended another PSA test in six months to see if the prescribed medication had helped.

Before my next appointment, I followed the doctor's recommendation by scheduling lab work and paid a visit to the local pharmacist to have the prescription filled. Completing the ten-day dose of medication, I had not felt any better down there and called the doctor's office to inform him. He responded by prescribing another dose of medication for what he believed was an inflamed prostate, and I followed his recommendation.

THE BIOPSY

Five or so months later I was back at the doctors' office for the result of my most recent PSA screening. The score had not decreased, instead, it was even higher, 6.9, in fact. This whole ordeal had gone on for over a year or so. Now, he was ready to perform a prostate biopsy on me. The doctor explained the procedure in his office and told me that I would lay on my side while he inserted an instrument into my rectum that was capable of injecting needles into the prostate in order to extract samples of tissue that would be sent to a laboratory for testing. After I agreed to the procedure, he directed me to an exam room where it was carried out, taking about 20 to 30 minutes. Afterwards, he informed me that the results would take approximately two weeks to come back.

At my next appointment, a month later, the doctor told me that he could not tell whether I did or did not have prostate cancer. I could not believe what I was hearing. *"What do you mean you cannot tell?" "Well,"* he said, *"I cannot definitively say whether you have cancer."*

Unsatisfied with his answer and lacking confidence in his ability to accurately diagnose my condition, I realized I had already risked enough with that doctor. So, I returned to my primary care provider, Dr. Maurice Bell, explained the situation, and asked for a second opinion, which he gladly offered.

A SECOND OPINION

In January of 2014, I had an appointment with a new urologist, Dr. Shahrad Aynehchi, MD, FACS who reviewed my medical file and history with me. He recommended that I have a second biopsy of the prostate to determine for the last time whether or not I had cancer. Concurring with his recommendation, the doctor performed the biopsy at his facility. During the procedure, I sensed a different level of skill and expertise in this new doctor as he manipulated the instrument, and felt confident that he knew what he was doing. After the biopsy, his nurse scheduled me for the next appointment in February to review the results.

A word about seeking a second opinion: While I'm not offering medical advice, I strongly encourage you not to hesitate if you feel the need to get one. In my case, I knew something wasn't quite right, so I trusted what my mind and body were telling me. I could feel that something was wrong in my pelvic region, and I needed to find out exactly what it was. I became my own best advocate and you can too.

CHAPTER SIX
Getting the News

The day had arrived—four o'clock on a Thursday afternoon. After waiting for what felt like the longest fifteen minutes of my life in the lobby, the nurse finally called me in. One thing I quickly noticed about this doctor was that he was a straight shooter, no nonsense. As I sat down in the chair, he got right to the point and told me that I had cancer. And not just any cancer—an "*extremely aggressive form of it*," to be exact.

Upon hearing the results, I was completely shocked. Sitting there speechless, my mouth wide open, I tried to speak but could not. The doctor suggested that I take a breath and try to relax. Moments later, gathering my breath and wits, I was able to speak. The first question I remember asking was whether he was certain, and the second question was when could he operate.

He told me that he was certain that I had cancer, then explained the types of medical procedures available to me, as well as his plan. He said, "*There is the traditional, open radical prostatectomy and the robotic procedure.*" During open surgery, a trained doctor and his staff would perform the procedure with instruments held in their hands. Usually, because the surgeon operates with his/her hands to remove the prostate and must make an incision to go through the bladder to access the prostate, men will most likely leak afterward. Generally, the incision to suture or close the wound to the bladder by hand will not be as precise, as opposed to the robotic procedure, where the capability of suturing will be more precise resulting in minimal or no leakage at all. Though the doctor would use the highest level of magnification available during the traditional procedure in addition to his or her level of skill and experience, there are no guarantees that a patient will not leak. He also assured me that he had already performed hundreds if not thousands of the traditional procedure, which was comforting to hear. The robotic procedure, new at the time, requires significant additional training to properly manipulate the robotic arms and instruments. A trained surgeon using the robotic platform must become highly proficient with it to achieve favorable outcomes and avoid complications. A physician will become proficient by performing hundreds if not thousands of operations. Physicians performing the robotic procedure without adequate training and experience could do more harm to a patient by improper manipulation due to unfamiliarity with the equipment.

After explaining the types of operations, he went into what I could expect afterwards. There may be side effects from the surgery and radiation treatment he had recommended. I may leak urine which would require wearing a pad and there was a possibility that I could become impotent. He kept talking for another fifteen or twenty seconds, but I did not hear a thing. Peeing on myself and not being able to have sex was all I heard before the ringing in my ears began. It was a good thing that I was already sitting down because the blows kept coming.

We talked about additional tests, such as Ultrasounds, C T Scans, and an MRI that I had to complete before his nurse could schedule me for surgery. He asked whether I had any questions, to which I had none. He patted me on the back and said, *"Don't worry, you're in good hands. I'll see you in a few weeks to a month for your procedure."*

I left his office carrying my self-esteem and ego in my hands. Somehow, I made it from the third floor of the doctor's office, out of the building, past the parking attendant, and into my car. Feeling the weight and burden of unwelcome news upon my shoulder, I started the car to make the long drive home.

And it truly was a long drive home. What normally would have been a 30 minute trip turned into about 3 hours. In the first hour of driving, I drove about twenty miles per hour less than the posted speed limit. In the second hour, I drove by my house circling the block repeatedly. Finally, I parked in the driveway and sat there for an hour thinking. I could not believe that I had cancer. How did I get it? Why me? What am I going to tell my wife and kids? How am I going to tell them?

Realizing that the family had not made it home themselves, there was a little more time to prepare. Gathering my thoughts, I decided I would say, "Honey, I need to talk to you. No honey, please sit down, I saw the doctor today and it was not good news."

An hour later, the three of them walked through the front door. My wife Anne and two sons, Jeremy and Tommy, ages 24 and 22. They had gone out together to pick up take-out for dinner. Placing the containers of food on the kitchen table, the boys went off to wash their hands and return to eat. I took that opportunity to separate my wife from them and guide her into a private room so that we could talk. I struggled to tell her what the doctor had told me, but I made it through. She was as shocked as I was and appeared devastated. Though she remained strong, she was compassionate and told me I had her support. Neither of us ate dinner that night. When the boys finished their meals, I spoke with them next. They seemed pretty shaken at first, but appeared to grasp the gravity of the situation. Dad was sick and needed an operation.

Everyone went off to bed that night to sleep in their respective rooms, but I needed to be alone. It was late, but I could not sleep. Sitting in our family room in the dark for hours, I searched through the day's events in the pages of my mind, trying to make sense of it all.

Soon, it was Friday morning and time to prepare for work. At work, I kept to myself as much as possible, making it through the day. Quitting time came and I set off for home.

A day or two later, I shared the news with my siblings, who came over to ask questions and offer their love, prayers, and support. *"Anything you need,"* each of them said. *"We are here for you no matter what."* I thanked them and told them that if something came up, I would let them know. Then one by one, each of them hugged me and walked out the front door.

Sleep did not come easy for several weeks. I remember sitting in a room alone each night for weeks. Using the glare emanating from the TV, I would sit in the family room staring at a clock on the wall wondering how long I might live. Wondering, what if surgery or radiation does not work? Was I ready to meet my maker? It was time to pray again. To ask God to calm my spirit and heal my body, and to prepare myself for whatever came next.

In between my sleepless nights and prayer meetings with God, I had completed all the necessary additional tests and screenings prior to the scheduled date for surgery. It was time to inform my supervisor that I had cancer and would be taking time off from work. The week before the scheduled surgery, I went into her office, sat down, and gave her the news. *"No problem,"* she said, *"we'll be here when you return." "Thanks for your support, Sergeant, I appreciate it,"* I responded.

With that box checked, I left work and headed home. When I arrived, I decided to research the procedure, with just days to go before having surgery. My doctor had given me two or three details to think about, but at the time, I was not focused. What was Open Radical Prostatectomy and Radiation therapy? What did each consist of? How long would each take? To satisfy my curiosity, I searched through YouTube videos about prostate cancer surgeries and radiation treatments.

After watching two videos of patients undergoing the open procedure, I got a general idea of what to expect. The surgery was lengthy, highly detailed, and invasive—affecting vital organs—and required a team of about three doctors, two technicians, and several other staff members. In contrast, the videos on radiation treatment were far less dramatic. It involved a radiologist, a technician, and a large machine used to position and treat the patient. I learned I would need to undergo radiation for approximately 39 consecutive weeks. With that information in hand, I felt more prepared for what lay ahead.

CHAPTER SEVEN
Surgery and Radiation

On an early Wednesday morning, in the spring of 2014, my wife and I arrived at the hospital to check me in. After a half hour wait, a nurse called me into a large room where there were other patients hidden behind curtains that served as partitions. Once inside my enclosed area, the nurse checked my vital signs. Minutes later, she gave me the infamous gown, which would expose my buttocks, a cap, and socks to put on before she returned. She had come back with a gurney, smiled, then asked me to "climb aboard" to which I obliged.

SURGERY

Soon after, I was on my way into the operating room where my doctor, an anesthesiologist, other doctors, and medical assistants stood by. Chatting briefly with me, my doctor told me, *"Don't worry you're in good hands, I'll see you in recovery."* The anesthesiologist gave me a spinal epidural and an IV (intravenous drip) with general anesthesia. Seven or eight hours later, I woke up in the recovery room. IV attached, medication flowing, regular blood pressure checks, and the best catered food in town. I could not be happier.

The doctor came by to check on me that evening to find that all was well. I had come through the surgery without any complications, he reported. He expressed optimism about removing all the cancer and stated that we would proceed as planned, which meant continuing recovery and in a couple of months, it would be time to begin radiation treatment.

A couple of days later, the doctor discharged me from the hospital and I went home to recover. In a week's time, I had a follow up visit with the doctor to monitor my progress. "*You're doing well,*" he said, "*remember to take it easy.*" I was eager to begin walking on the treadmill, about a mile or two for exercise. His nurse scheduled me for another visit with the doctor in a month to check the progress and talk about the upcoming treatment.

At my next appointment, the doctor explained that it was necessary for me to have and complete a specific number of targeted radiation treatments. He referred me to a doctor of radiology to make my first appointment.

RADIATION

Following his instruction, I planned to see the next doctor. She turned out to be extremely knowledgeable, pleasant, and caring. There were two additional tests I would need to undergo prior to the start of treatment. Then she discussed her plan of action, including what I should expect during treatment, and how my progress would be monitored.

If memory serves me correctly, I went twice a week for about 39 weeks. Following the doctor's and technicians' instructions, each time I went for an appointment, I entered a room that housed one of the largest machines I had ever seen. It had a large round glaze donut shaped appearance with about an 8 foot-long padded table in its center. As I lay on the table, the technician guided me into the precise position for each targeted strike, then slid me and the table into the center of the machine. Once in position, the staff member left the room, peered through a window, then activated the machine. She would speak to me using a P. A. system telling me when to breathe in, hold my breath, and when to exhale.

Every time I had to endure one of those treatments, it felt like the lone-liest time of my life. It is something that each of us in need of radiation therapy must experience alone. No one could be in the room with me. Not even my wife. It reminded me of the song by Harry Nilsson, *"One is the loneliest number."* The number one stands alone, just as a patient does during radiation treatment.

Meeting with the radiologist periodically, she would update my prog-ress, and asked how I thought things were going and whether I had any questions. My usual reply was I'm doing fine, and I do not have any questions. Remembering an episode of diarrhea, I was too embar-rassed to discuss it with her, so I let it go. On my last visit with the doc-tor, I asked if diarrhea was a side effect of the treatment, to which the doctor replied, *"yes."* Well, imagine that. Who would have thought? She then assured me that the therapy was a success and that my body had responded well. Thanking the doctor for what she and her staff had done, we parted ways.

I was grateful to have completed both surgery and radiation—and even more thankful to be alive. I'm especially thankful that I didn't ac-cept the inconclusive results from the first urologist and that I chose to seek a second opinion. I owe a deep debt of gratitude to my urologist, Dr. Aynehchi, not only for the life-saving surgery he performed but also for his editorial contributions to this handbook. Without him and the good Lord, I wouldn't be here sharing my story or offering guidance on managing urinary incontinence (leakage) and erectile dysfunction (impotence).

CHAPTER EIGHT
The Realization

With surgery and radiation treatment under my belt, I began to reflect on what my urologist had said and what my wife and I went through in the first few weeks or so after surgery. The side effects were real. The reality of constantly leaking urine and erectile dysfunction are true. I left the hospital wearing a urinary collection bag and a medical drain. The urinary collection bag was the only one I had and I wore it religiously, emptying it often. We became good friends. That bag and me.

There was however, a down side that came along with wearing that urinary collection bag as well as the medical drain. At some point during the operation while I was asleep, a catheter was inserted into my privates to aid in urination during and after the procedure and a drain was attached inside my body for any fluid build up. Upon being discharged from the hospital, I was given aftercare instructions. I was to apply ice to the penis for about 20 minutes at a time throughout the day for the next few days to reduce swelling and to empty the contents of the drain as needed.

Following the instructions religiously, the swelling had gone away, but an intense burning sensation arrived every time I would urinate through that catheter and into the urinary collection bag. It made me not want to urinate at all, but of course that was not possible. So, I had to suffer through that unpleasantry for about 3 or 4 days until my next appointment with the urologist who would remove the catheter and also the medical drain that had been attached inside my body to capture any fluid build-up from the surgical procedure.

Removing both the catheter and the drain were slightly painful when the time had come. I was instructed to take a deep breath during each extraction, then exhale and it was over. These two details, the good doctor had not advised me of on the day that he explained the types of treatments he recommended and their potential side effects that I could expect. So, I thought I would share those juicy tidbits with you, not that they are something for you to look forward to.

In the first 4 weeks after the surgery, my wife decided that it was necessary to evaluate the veracity of my doctor's claim that I could become impotent. So, one night she slipped into an amazing night gown that accentuated her wares, then she paraded them in front of me. Normally, that would result in Sha-boing time for me, but Mr. TJ never woke up. Sadly, my wife had confirmed what I already knew, no boom, boom would be happening. She was frustrated because I could not perform, and because I was unable to have an erection, I was extremely discouraged.

That's why it's so important for you and your partner to be on the same page—emotionally, physically, and in terms of expectations. If you are awaiting results of a prostate biopsy, invite your spouse or significant other to attend the appointment with you. That way, if you are diagnosed with prostate cancer, the doctor will explain all the potential side effects and any risks associated with surgery, radiation, and recovery, and your loved one will be there to hear it and take it all in with you. In my case, I hadn't even told my wife about my biopsy, I didn't want to worry her if there would be no reason to.

The healing process had barely begun. It was too soon to expect that I would be ready to perform, or if I even could perform. She may have been thinking that I was still my old self, you know, business as usual. The doctor had told me that he would do his best during the surgery to preserve the surrounding nerves when removing the prostate, stating that, *"these nerves travel close to the prostate on either side and can easily be damaged if the cancer is encroaching on them."* He felt that a nerve sparing technique would afford me the best chance at maintaining potency. *"However,"* he added, *"even with full preservation of the nerves, there is no guarantee that they will fully function after surgery."*

I am happy to say that he was right to use the nerve sparing technique. Because with God's blessing and the surgeon's expertise, I was able to regain the satisfactory function of that part of my anatomy with the assistance of modern medicine. Assistance that I never thought in a million years I would need.

Even though the doctor had spoken to me about leaking urine and becoming impotent after surgery and/or radiation, those concerns had not registered foremost in my mind. I was still recovering from the whole reality of having cancer. I had given little thought, if any, to the changes in life circumstances I would face.

There were no thoughts about how I would get around town, work, or travel, until the phone rang. My supervisor. *"TJ, It's Mick. You're out of sick time and you're due back to work on Monday morning. Okay?"* Not knowing what else to say, I said, *"okay,"* and that I would be there.

When I hung up the phone, I thought, what am I going to do? It was Friday afternoon with Monday morning fast approaching. I had to produce a plan to deal with the problem of leaking urine so that I could go back to work.

CHAPTER NINE
The Guide

MANAGING URINARY INCONTINENCE AND IMPOTENCE

As I mentioned earlier, urinary leakage and the inability to achieve or maintain an erection are common side effects of prostate cancer surgery and/or radiation. To manage the leakage, I began an online search for reliable, discreet products designed for personal use. My goal was to find solutions from reputable companies that would allow me to manage incontinence on my own—without the need for additional surgery. I chose a self-management approach to take control of this aspect of my recovery.

My urologist had informed me "of a surgical alternative," but I was not inclined to try it because of the potential risks involved, which we will identify later in the next section.

While researching male incontinence products, I discovered several self-help options for managing urinary leakage at work, while traveling, or at home—specifically, male guards and the Afex® system.

MANAGING URINARY INCONTINENCE
Self-Management

- Depend®, Guards for men. Available online and in local stores.
- The Afex® Management system for male incontinence, currently available at Arcusmed.com/shop, Amazon, and through other vendors. The system consists of specifically designed underwear, a specially designed funnel, a collection unit, a canister, and cleaning solvent. The user of the funnel and collection unit should clean them daily after each use and it should last about thirty days before replacement is needed. You may purchase each item separately or as a kit. Please follow the manufacturer's instructions for use and cleaning. Note that the funnel is designed to connect to the collection bag by twisting them together. After repeated application the connection might begin to stick and may require some lubrication to operate smoothly.

With the discovery of these two products, the Depend® pads and the incontinence system, I was ready to report to work Monday morning. I expedited the delivery of the system for that weekend so that there was time to familiarize myself with its use the coming week. My wife picked up a couple of packages of the Depend® guards from a local Walmart.

I developed a system of alternating use of the two products daily or weekly for about 3 years until retiring in 2017. Through trial and error, on the days when I wore pads, I learned to change them once per hour due to potential saturation. Oversaturation would lead to a wardrobe malfunction, which would result in the need to change clothes or undergarments worn. Another discovery revealed that the more liquid I drank, the more I would leak, even while wearing a pad or device. So, it was important to find a balance. It is also necessary to drain or empty the urinary collection bag at least once per hour or as often as needed.

With increasing amounts of fluid, the bag can become weighted. I remember Dr. Aynehchi explained some other reasons for urine leakage after treatment. He said, *"Sometimes it's minor or moderate but in other cases, it can be severe—especially during activities like sitting, standing, coughing, laughing, sneezing, walking, running, or jumping."* In my case, the leakage is more severe. This explains the amount of urine that can accumulate over time and why access to a restroom is essential. You should make access to a restroom part of your daily plan— whether you're out and about or driving, especially on longer trips.

Use of either the pads or the incontinence system each had their drawbacks. For the pads, there was the unmistakable odor of urine that not only I was able to sense but also anyone else standing in proximity to me. If or when the collection bag filled to about two hundred milliliters, I would often hear a swishing sound as I walked. Hearing that sound would immediately prompt me to empty it.

Another realization I had about wearing a urinary collection bag at work between 2014 and 2017 was the potential risk it posed—not just to me, but to my employer. Because I worked in law enforcement, there was always the possibility of getting into a physical altercation with a suspect or member of the public. If a scuffle had occurred while I was wearing the collection bag, it could have burst, potentially spilling its contents on me or someone else—a scenario that would've been catastrophic for all involved. Thankfully, I was never in such a situation during that time. Looking back, I would not recommend wearing a collection bag in high-risk or physically active environments.

By 2018, I discovered other options that could be used alongside male pads or guards, such as the Pacey Cuff or the Virth Incontinence Clamp. If you're considering either of these, be sure to read and follow the manufacturers' instructions carefully. These devices take some getting used to, so patience and practice are essential. I recommend wearing the cuff or clamp for no more than one hour at a time as you acclimate—and never while sleeping. Always keep track of how long you've worn it. Even though I've experienced wardrobe malfunctions using both devices—even within the recommended time—they've still proven to be worthwhile investments. Just be sure to have backup supplies on hand, as listed in the following sections, for when you're not using the cuff or clamp.

The Pacey Cuff is available in small, medium, and large sizes that should accommodate most men and the Virth Clamp provides 3 varied sizes to choose from to fit most men as well. Both require little maintenance for upkeep. You will affix either the cuff or clamp around the circumference of the male appendage. Consider taking care not to pinch yourself during its application. You should also use caution if you are wearing either the Cuff or Clamp while driving. Things to consider are, the duration of your trip, time of day, traffic congestion, traffic delays, or being involved in a traffic collision. Remember the cuff and clamp are restricting or controlling the flow of leakage while worn and as time passes, pressure builds, and so will the urge to relieve yourself. You might consider wearing a pad while driving, then switching to the cuff or clamp with a pad after reaching your destination. More about these devices in the upcoming list of items you might consider wearing while at work to control the flow of urine.

LIST OF ITEMS FOR WORK

Below is a list of products I used while working, along with additional items I discovered along the way. These proved invaluable, especially when I was away from home:

- **Depend® Disposable Male Pads** – Replenish as needed. Available online and in stores. I often kept extra pads tucked in my socks for convenience. Occasionally, I wore two pads for extra protection, though this did not prevent potential malfunctions.Wear the pad(s) with Wearever® reusable underwear.
- **Pacey Cuff (2)** – A device that controls the flow of urine. Replace

quarterly. Available at paceycuff.com, Amazon, or other vendors.

- **Virth Incontinence Clamps (2)** – Another urinary-control device. Replace quarterly. Available at Amazon and other vendors.
- **Wearever® Men's Reusable Incontinence Underwear** – Designed with a padded front. Best worn with a supporter and pad, or a cuff/clamp and pad. Available at MyWearever.com or Amazon.
- **Male Athletic Supporters** – Used in combination with pads and underwear. Available online or in stores.
- **Disposable Baby Wipes (e.g., Huggies® or Dude Wipes®)** – For freshening up the pelvic region.
- **Extra Uniform/Work Pants** – To have on hand in case of wardrobe malfunctions during work hours.
- **Extra Casual Pants or Shorts** – For commuting or unplanned accidents.
- **Plastic Bags** – For storing soiled garments until you return home.
- **Backpack** – To carry and organize your daily incontinence supplies.

LIST OF ITEMS FOR TRAVEL

Whether traveling for work or leisure, the following items helped me maintain comfort and hygiene:

- **Depend® Disposable Male Pads** – Replenish as needed. Extra pads can be stored in socks for convenience in conjunction with Wearever® underwear.
- **Afex® Male Urinary Incontinence Unit** – *Note: I do not recommend wearing the collection bag through airport security. Instead, wear a pad or clamp and change afterward if needed.*
- **Pacey Cuff or Virth Clamp (plus a backup)** – Follow all manufacturer instructions. Use with reusable underwear and a pad. Supporter optional.
- **Wearever® Men's Reusable Underwear** – Worn with pad and op-

tionally with a supporter.

- **Athletic Supporters (Weekly Supply)** – Helps keep the penis aligned with the pad to help contain leaks.
- **Disposable Baby Wipes** – Carry a package or place two folded wipes in a small zip-lock bag and store them in your sock when traveling.
- **Change of Clothing** – Always have backup clothing in case of leaks.
- **Plastic Bags** – For soiled garments and other refuse.
- **Small Travel Bucket** – For storing cleaning supplies such as bleach, funnel, and the collection unit.
- **Hand Towels** – Use when stepping out of hotel showers.
- **Depend® Disposable Underwear** – Worn with a supporter during exercise. Pad optional.
- **Backpack** – For carrying all travel supplies.

LIST OF ITEMS FOR HOME

The following are the products I used daily at home to manage incontinence with comfort and peace of mind:

- **Depend® Disposable Male Pads** – Replenish as needed. You may double up pads (replace the top one after an hour), though this won't guarantee prevention of a malfunction.
- **Depend® Disposable Underwear** – Especially useful during physical activity or workouts.
- **Pacey Cuffs (2) or Virth Clamps (2)** – Choose the device that works best for you. *Note: Leakage may occur with either device. This could mean it's time to tighten one notch or replace the product. Do not wear it beyond one hour and never sleep while wearing it.*
- **Wearever® Men's Reusable Underwear (Weekly Supply)** – Worn with pads and optionally with a supporter during the day and while sleeping.
- **Athletic Supporters** – Helps keep the penis in position to avoid

56

leaks outside the pad. Use it with underwear and pads.

- **Disposable Baby Wipes** – Keep on hand for quick clean-ups during pad changes.

Now that you have gained insight into the availability of Male Incontinence products on the market for self-management, you may be able to set your mind at ease. You can still work, travel, and play knowing that with a plan you will be ready for just about anything. As you read through the list of items for daily use, whether it be for work, travel, or play, you may notice an overlapping of products. There is no need to double or triple procurement of these products, such as the athletic supporters, cuffs, clamps, wipes, or reusable underwear, because they may be repurposed when using a different list, but after a month or two, you will need to replenish some items as needed.

MANAGEMENT OF URINARY INCONTINENCE
Medical/Surgical Approach

During one of my post prostate surgery appointments with the urologist, Dr. Aynehchi discussed the possibility of me undergoing a medical or surgical procedure for a more permanent solution to urinary incontinence. He suggested that after my body had a couple of months to heal, that I might be interested in having him medically insert an artificial urinary sphincter (AUS) into my pelvic region to control or prevent leakage. To urinate, I would manually activate it. He went on to explain that after he performed the procedure on a subject, the patient may or may not benefit from it.

ADVANTAGES OF AN ARTIFICIAL URINARY SPHINCTER

- Ability to control, slow, or prevent urinary leakage.
- If you no longer leak, you may resume a normal quality of life.
- No need to limit or monitor the quantity of fluids consumed each day.
- No need to purchase and wear pads, cuffs, clamps, or bags.

- No need for frequent restroom breaks.
- If leakage is minimal, you may be able to reduce the quantity of products needed for daily use.
- Reduced financial expense.
- Minimal or no wardrobe malfunctions, if any.

DISADVANTAGES OF AN ARTIFICIAL URINARY SPHINCTER

- The procedure was ineffective.
- The procedure could make leakage worse.
- The procedure could cause an infection.
- Recovery period.
- Revision of the procedure.
- You must manipulate a mechanism to urinate.

I wasn't ready to make a decision, so I went on managing my urinary incontinence myself.

In October of 2023, I began seeing a new urologist, Dr. Howard Aubert, MD. After an initial evaluation and medical screening, he explained that managing my urinary incontinence could better be addressed by also undergoing a medical procedure, but one called bulking. A new concept, developed for women around 2018, that has since been adapted for men. It offers those injected with a gel into a specific area of their body another option for treating urinary incontinence. The doctor went on to identify the advantages and disadvantages of the procedure. They are as follows:

ADVANTAGES OF BULKING

- Ability to control or prevent urinary leakage.
- Performed in the doctor's office in about 20 minutes.
- Less invasive than alternative procedures.

- Faster recovery.
- If successful, you will regain an improved quality of life.
- Infrequent restroom trips.
- Fewer wardrobe malfunctions, if any.
- Minimal need for a backup plan or supplies.
- Cost savings.

DISADVANTAGES OF BULKING

- The procedure did not work.
- The physician used insufficient gel resulting in a revision of the procedure.
- An infection may occur.
- The procedure may inflame or cause additional urinary leakage.
- May result in additional heartache, inconvenience, and expense.
- Physicians have reported additional side effects.

After meeting with both doctors and discussing the pros and cons of each procedure, I ultimately decided against both options. My decision was primarily based on the potential risks of infection, revision, or worsening the current issue with leakage. However, you may be more willing to accept these risks if you feel the potential benefits outweigh them. Ultimately, each of us must weigh the facts, risks, and possible outcomes to make an informed decision that feels right for our individual situation.

MANAGING IMPOTENCE

If you have had either prostate cancer surgery or radiation treatment, chances are you may experience erectile dysfunction, whether it be partial or complete impotence. Remember, impotence is a known potential side effect that men may suffer from for the rest of their lives.

Dr. Aynehchi explained it in terms that I could understand, "*During prostate surgery and/or radiation treatment, the possibility exists for damage to the nerves that help with erections. Treatment relative to the male anatomy in the pelvic region could render most men partially or completely impotent."* Yet, he assured me that he would do his utmost best to preserve the neurovascular bundles during the surgery, to afford me the best chance in recovery of my sexual function. As I mentioned earlier, he was able to preserve enough of the nerves in that region by using a nerve-sparing technique. Fortunately, the cancer had not spread to those areas. Those two factors turned out to be a blessing, allowing me to regain satisfactory sexual function with the help of medication. Consistent use of the prescribed medication has been key in managing erectile dysfunction effectively.

If you've undergone prostate surgery or radiation treatment, you may find yourself in a similar situation. Perhaps your doctor used a nerve-sparing technique, and the cancer had not spread to the surrounding nerves. Thanks to your physician's efforts, you may now be only partially impotent. If you've been prescribed a medication like Viagra® and it's working well, you're already on the path to effectively managing erectile dysfunction.

Being able to share intimate moments with your significant other is deeply important. If you're fortunate enough to have some functional recovery—and medication can help enhance that experience—then following your doctor's advice can go a long way toward improving your quality of life.

Now there are others whose doctors have recently diagnosed them with prostate cancer who may not have known about the potential side effects of surgery and radiation therapy, but now have gained insight into them. So, each of you, with additional information on the relevant issues, can more effectively discuss with your doctor or urologist how to best address a treatment plan going forward.

On the other hand, some individuals may have undergone surgery and/or radiation therapy but, due to a lack of insurance, no longer have access to a doctor or treating urologist. As a result, you may not be able to obtain a prescription for Viagra® or similar medication, even if a previous doctor diagnosed you as partially impotent.

Fortunately, there are reputable online providers that offer prescribed medications for erectile dysfunction. If eligible, you may be able to receive a prescription through a virtual consultation. Below is a list of online sources that provide these services.

MANAGING IMPOTENCE WITH MEDICATION

- Sildenafil generic for Viagra® taken regularly as prescribed.
- Ro.co/sparks
- Hims.com/erectile-dysfunction
  https://www.hims.com/

CONCLUSION

It is my sincere hope that you've found the information in this handbook helpful and meaningful. Since being diagnosed with prostate cancer in 2014, I've undergone both surgery and radiation—experiences that profoundly changed my life. As a survivor, I've learned—through trial, error, and persistence—how to manage the side effects of urinary incontinence without relying on further medical or surgical interventions.

You, of course, will need to work closely with your healthcare provider to weigh the pros and cons of available options and decide what path is best for you. But the purpose of this handbook is to remove as much guesswork as possible by sharing what I've learned and what has worked for me. I encourage you to explore the self-management plans and product lists I've included—they've been invaluable in improving my quality of life, and they may help you as well.

This, in essence, is my story: a career in law enforcement that likely led to certain exposures and, ultimately, a diagnosis of prostate cancer. Thankfully, timely medical attention and the right support made all the difference. Today, my doctor and I continue to monitor my PSA levels every six months, staying vigilant for any signs of recurrence. And with that, I move forward—grateful, informed, and hopeful.

MESSAGES FROM PROSTATE CANCER SURVIVORS

March 26, 2025

I went to my doctor for my annual physical. My blood work discovered my PSA at 7.0. I had developed prostate cancer. My doctor and I discussed my options, so I decided to have surgery to remove the prostate. After additional testing we discovered my potassium was low, and after several more weeks the potassium level had not increased. I then elected to have radiation treatments. There were 20 treatments in all. Now that the treatments are over, I am having hot flashes and fatigue, and must have check-ups every three months. With the support of family and friends, it made the process much easier. With the treatments over at age 63, life is back to normal.

-Anonymous

March 29, 2025

Shock, disbelief, and anxiety gripped my thoughts when I received the news that I had prostate cancer. This was in the beginning of 2020, a time when the world was dealing with the emergence of the deadly COVID- 19 disease. My doctor and I had been monitoring my PSA levels over the years, noting the increase from 2.9 in 2015 to 4.2 in March of 2019, and then 5.4 in December of the same year. In addition to these changing numbers, I was experiencing frequent urination, which prompted my doctor to recommend a biopsy.

In January of 2020, I underwent the biopsy, and by February, the results confirmed what I dreaded to hear, "You have prostate cancer." Out of the 12 cores sampled, four were positive. My Gleason score was 3+3 in three cores and 4+3 in the other. My doctor was optimistic with the results though, believing that we had caught the cancer early enough to achieve a positive outcome. His optimism helped ease some of my anxiety, because I had a sister and brother die in 2007 from complications of metastatic colon cancer.

In March, I discussed treatment options with my oncologists. I spent much time in prayer, had numerous conversations with my wife and other men who had experienced prostate cancer. In addition, my sister who is both a doctor and a breast cancer survivor, offered invaluable advice. She shared that in her experience as a doctor and cancer patient, cancer tends to be more aggressive in Black individuals compared to other nationalities. Consequently, she suggested that it would be best to take the most aggressive approach. Although it was a difficult decision, I chose to have my prostate removed. The procedure was called a robot assisted Laparoscopic Radical Prostatectomy. This decision has turned out for the good. The cancer had not escaped the margins, and it allowed me to avoid chemotherapy and radiation, which was a tremendous relief. I like my grey hair!

Throughout this journey, my faith and support system were my strength. My wife and children were a constant source of encouragement, helping me stay positive despite the challenges. The surgery itself was tough, and dealing with the catheter and painful urination post-surgery was particularly challenging. I also had a severe tingling in my left leg that lasted over a year. The doctor said that it could have been nerve damage because of the position (inverted) I was placed in during the surgical procedure.
After the surgery, I remained optimistic despite having leakage and some erectile challenges. My doctor offered Sildenafil as an option, but it didn't

work, and an injection which improves erection. The initial aftermath was difficult to deal with, but knowing that the cancer had been caught early and eradicated kept me motivated.

My experience was difficult and very challenging at times, and I would not wish it on anyone. What has been reinforced is my belief in the importance of regular health check-ups, proper diet, regular exercise, and a strong support system. I have been able to continue living with no regrets with my decision. I would do it the same way if I had to do it over again.

Grace to you,

Anonymous, 67

ACKNOWLEDGEMENTS

Without a doubt, I owe special thanks to my wife Erika, for being thoughtful, patient, and considerate of me during the planning, research, drafting, writing, and completion of this handbook. She also took the time to read through many paragraphs and gently offered her input. I love you dearly and look forward to your quiet spirit and insightful inspiration at the advent of my next book.

Eternally yours,
Your loving husband, Taryton.

———————

A very special thanks to my former urologist and surgeon, Dr. Shahrad Aynehchi, MD. Your knowledge, training, experience, life saving surgery, and editorial contributions to this handbook are unparalleled. Thank you, Dr. Aynehchi, for the knowledge and skills you demonstrated during the performance of my prostate biopsy for a second opinion, in which you found the aggressive cancer that led to surgery and radiation treatment. I owe you a debt of gratitude in more ways than one.

Thanks again, Dr. Aynehchi,
Your grateful patient, Taryton.

SOURCES

THE PATHWAYS OF EXPOSURE

Diesel Exhaust, PAHs, and PFAS, U. S. cities that hire dual fire/police agencies

McCammon, Jane Brown, William D. Wagner, David H. Groth, G Kent Hatfield, Vanessa L. Becks, Ruth E. Grubbs, Anne C. Hamilton, et al. "Carcinogenic Effects of Exposure to Diesel Exhaust (88-116)." Edited by Laurence D. Reed. *Centers for Disease Control and Prevention*, June 6, 2014. Diesel Exposure at Work

Wardoyo, Arinto Y. P., Unggul P. Juswono, and Johan A. E. Noor. "How Exposure to Ultrafine and Fine Particles of Car Smoke Can Alter Erythrocyte Forms of Male Mice". Polish Journal of Environmental Studies 28 no. 4 (2019): 2901-2910. doi:10.15244/pjoes/94047.
"Niosh Potential Occupational Carcinogens." Centers for Disease Control and Prevention, Centers for Disease Control and Prevention, 17 Oct. 2018, www.cdc.gov/niosh/npg/nengapdxa.html.

"CDC - NIOSH Pocket Guide to Chemical Hazards - Carbon Black." Centers for Disease Control and Prevention, October 30, 2019. https://www.cdc.gov/niosh/npg/npgd0102.html.

"Polycyclic Aromatic Hydrocarbons (Pahs)." Centers for Disease Control and Prevention, August 28, 2014. https://wwwn.cdc.gov/TSP/PHS/PHS.aspx?phsid=120&toxid=25.

Polycyclic aromatic hydrocarbons (pahs) | toxicological profile | Atsdr. Accessed March 16, 2025. https://wwwn.cdc.gov/TSP/ToxProfiles/Tox-Profiles.aspx?id=122&tid=25.

Seidler A;Heiskel H;Bickeböller R;Elsner. G. "Association between Diesel Exposure at Work and Prostate Cancer." Scandinavian journal of work, environment & health, December 24, 1998. (6): 486-94. Doi: 10.5271/sjweh.373. PMID: 9988091

Firefighter's Cancer
Dodd, Johnny. "Firefighter's Cancer Leads Wife to Discovery of Toxic Gear Killing Heroes across U.S.: 'It's Infuriating.'" Peoplemag, December 27, 2023.
https://people.com/firefighters-cancer-leads-wife-to-discovery-of-toxic-gear-8420205.

Per-and Polyfluoroalkyl Substances
NIOSH. "Pfas." Centers for Disease Control and Prevention, September 15, 2022.
https://www.cdc.gov/niosh/topics/pfas/default.html.

us cities with dual fire/police agencies-Google Search
https://portal.cops.usdoj.gov/resourcecenter/content.ashx/cops-348-pub.pdf

RESOURCES

Agency for Toxic Substances and Disease Registry (ATSDR)
U.S Department of Health and Human Services
1600 Clifton Rd
Atlanta, GA, 30329
1-800-232-4636
www.atsdr.cdc.gov

Centers for Disease Control and Prevention (CDC)
1600 Clifton Rd.
Atlanta, GA 30329
1-800-232-4636
www.cdc.gov

U. S. Department of Health and Human Services (DHHS)
HHS Headquarters
200 Independence Avenue, S.W.
Washington, D.C. 20201
1-877-696-6775
www.hhs.gov

Division of Standards Development and Technology Transfer
Publications Dissemination, (DSDTT)
National Institute for Occupational Safety and Health
4676 Columbia Parkway
Cincinnati, Ohio 45226

1-513-841-4287
www.cdc.gov

National Biomonitoring Program (NBP)
Mailing address
National Biomonitoring Program
Division of Laboratory Sciences
Mail Stop F-204770
Buford Highway, N E
Atlanta, GA 30341-3724
1-800-232-4636
www.cdc.gov/biomonitoring/contact-us/index.html

National Institute for Occupational Safety and Health (NIOSH)
400 7th St. SW
Suite 5W
Washington, D C, 20024
1-800-232-4636
www.cdc.gov/niosh

Polish Journal of Environmental Studies
"HARD" Publishing Company s.c.
Jerzy Radecki, Hanna Radecka, Dorota Radecka
WENGRIS 71 Street
10-765 OLSZTYN
POLAND
https://www.pjoes.com

INCONTINENCE/IMPOTENCE RESOURCES, MEDICATIONS AND DEVICES

Acquisition of Incontinence Products online, i.e., pads, clamps, etc....
www.amazon.com
Afex® Male Urinary Incontinence Unit
www.arcusmedical.com

Artificial Urinary Sphincter
See urologist for details

Athletic Supporters
Can be acquired online and various retailers

Bulking
See urologist for details

Depend® Disposable Underwear
Available at various retailers

Depend® Male Guards
May be purchased at various retailers

Erectile Dysfunction
Obtain prescription where applicable, i.e., Ro.com/sparks

Pacey Cuff
Urethral control device www.pacdycuff.com

Wearever® Reusable Underwear
Available at www.mywearever.com or www.amazon.com

Virth Incontinence Clamp
Can be acquired online at www.amazon.com

INDEX

GLOSSARY

Adam-12- A 1960's Law enforcement television show.

Afex® Male Urinary Incontinence System- A male incontinence system designed to manage the collection of urine.

Agency for Toxic Substances and Disease Registration (ATSDR)- A Federal health affiliate within the United States Government's Department of Health and Human Services.

Anesthesiologist- A trained doctor or medical professional who specializes in the administration of specific medications provided to patients undergoing surgical procedures. The medication given may render a person unconscious to reduce or minimize the awareness of pain or discomfort.

Arcus® Medical LLC/ Arcus Medical.com- A company headquartered in Charlotte, North Carolina that designs, manufactures, and sells incontinence products.

Artificial Urinary Sphincter- A surgically inserted device designed to address medium to excessive urinary incontinence or leakage.

Athletic Supporter- A supportive item of clothing worn by men, usually during sports activities, made of material capable of expanding or contracting to its original position.

Biopsy- A type of medical procedure performed by a medical professional who will extract a sample of tissue from a person to determine the existence or degree of disease in the body.

Bitumen- A black thick or sticky petroleum substance that may be hard or free flowing such as water or oil.

Black Top- A type of material commonly used as the top layer on many roads or highways.

Blood Pressure- The intensity of the blood in the cardiovascular system is usually measured for determination in relation to the power and caliber of heartbeat and the girth and flexibility of the arterial walls.

Blood Work- A scientific or systematic process of evaluating one or more samples of blood. Usually, to search for illness.

Bulking- An in-office medical procedure performed by a urologist. He or she may inject specific or targeted amounts of a gel or substance into a male or female urethra to control or manage urinary incontinence.

Cancer- A disorder that occurs in an area of a person's body where some normal cells have become abnormal and may expand into other areas within the body.

Carbon Black- A toxin found in polycyclic aromatic hydrocarbons. (PAHs)

Carcinogen- A type of medium that possesses the ability to advance the growth of cancer, such as a synthetic chemical.

Catheter- A slender straw like hose used to facilitate the ingress and egress of bodily liquids or medications.

Centers for Disease Control and Prevention (CDC)- It is the Countries public health agency for the United States of America. A Federal agency affiliated within the Department of Health and Human Services.

Computed Tomography Scan (CT scan)- A medical procedure that allows trained professionals to produce visualizations of a subject's internal body parts.

Craftsman Home- A distinctively designed type of home dating back to the American craftsman movement that began in the 1900's.

Department of Health and Human Services (DHHS)- An agency of the United States of America. Its mission is to improve the overall health of the American public.

Depend® Disposable Underwear- A single use disposable undergarment worn by men or women who may suffer from incontinence.

Depend® Guards- A single use pad worn by men designed to absorb leaking urine.

Diagnosis- An examination by a medical or dental professional of a patient's complaint of discomfort to determine the cause of their problem (s).

Diesel Exhaust- Fumes created as result of the activation of a diesel motor and include the production of airborne contaminants.

Division of Standards and Technology Transfer (DSDTT)- Is an organization within the United States Government that facilitates a network of documents for the research, development, and transfer of reports among several federal laboratories.

Doctor of Radiology- A licensed medical professional who holds a medical degree. He or she has received the necessary training and experience to read, diagnose, and treat patients after examining a captured image.

Dude Wipes®- Wipes developed for men's personal use or hygiene.

Epidermal Layer- The visible or exposed layer of a person's skin.

Erectile Dysfunction- Usually when a male is unable to have or continue to have an erection strong enough to have sex.

Exhaust Emission(s)- A combination of various gases or fumes that contain specks flowing from an automobile while the motor is on.

Extremely Superior Particles of Matter- Particles of matter that are extremely small.

Firefighter- A person who has received training and experience in fire suppression to help save lives and protect property from being harmed or destroyed.

Firefighting Froth- A specific type of chemical that produces bubbles used to arrest fire.

Firefighting Profession- An occupation charged with the task of preventing, managing, and extinguishing fire.

Fireman's Protective Apparel- Commonly known as turnout gear, it is composed of material to protect the wearer from various heat sources, flashes of intense heat, and risks from holes or cuts.

Fluid Build Up- The collection of liquid matter, blood, or other fluids that may gather in an internal body part, body pocket, or injury site of the body.

Fossil Fuel- Used to create energy, they are a group of chemicals composed of hydrogen and carbon.

Freight Cycle- The allocation of time a circuit remains activated in relation to the time it is terminated.

General anesthesia- The process of medically causing a person to lose awareness of their senses usually during most surgical procedures.

Gun-Belt- A gun belt or utility belt usually made of leather or canvas material is designed to accommodate the user's attached weapon and other pertinent equipment.

Gurney- An apparatus capable of shifting into a horizontal or semi-vertical position such as a chair. Often used to transport people who may or may not be incapacitated.

Hims- An online internet portal that enables men to confidentially consult with a health care provider for assistance related to their sexual health and well-being.

Huggies® Baby Wipes- Developed to cleanse a person's pelvic region, usually due to soiled underwear or diapers.

Impotence- The inability of a male to have or keep an erection.

Inflammation- The body's reaction to injury or other harm it is exposed to and may present itself by signs of pain, swelling, or other types of manifestations.

Intravenous Drip (IV)- The process of administering the necessary liquids, medical substances, or foods by injection into a vein in the body.

Laboratory- A specially equipped facility designed to conduct tests, studies, instruction, or create medications or other compounds.

Law Enforcement Officer- A person employed and empowered by a government or municipality to uphold, enforce, and investigate persons suspected of committing crimes.

Less Superior Particles of Matter- Particles of matter that are larger than minute particles.

Magnetic Resonance Imaging (MRI)- A method of examining the internal organs and systems of a person's anatomy using a combination of magnets and radio frequencies to form an image doctors can evaluate.

Male Incontinence Products- Products that have been designed specifically for men to help manage or control urinary incontinence.

Medical Drain-A straw like medical conduit introduced into the site of an incision during an operation to permit the unrestricted release of body fluids that might collect while a patient recovers from a surgical procedure.

Medical / Surgical Approach-Treatments usually performed by a trained and experienced urologist to treat men or women suffering from urinary incontinence.

Medication- A prescribed medical substance for the treatment of an illness or injury that will often improve a patient's symptoms or discomfort.

National Biomonitoring Program (NBP)- Observes, discovers, and collects samples of potentially harmful substances in the atmosphere for evaluation and analysis.

National Institute for Occupational Safety and Health (NIOSH)- NIOSH is affiliated with the Centers for Disease Control and Prevention (CDC), under the umbrella of the Department of Health and Human Services.

Nerves- A collection of threads that upon stimulation send signals to various areas of the body.

Nerve Sparing- A method that some skilled surgeons employ during surgery to preserve or limit any damage or potential damage to the integrity of the nerve bundles.

Neurovascular Bundles- An arrangement or structure that ties nerves, veins, and other fibrous systems with other matter enabling them to move through the body.

Non-Diesel Engine- A motor vehicle that has been equipped with an internal combustion engine that requires petroleum or common forms of gasoline as fuel to operate.

Noxious Fumes- Extremely toxic or hazardous chemicals that can be detrimental to humans or animals.

Occupational and Environmental Hazards- They are an array of dangers that employers or employees may be exposed to in the workplace.

Open Radical Prostatectomy- A surgical treatment that many trained surgeons or urologists perform to extract the male prostate gland.

Pacey Cuff- A device developed for men who suffer from urinary incontinence.

Pad- A soft material designed to absorb leaking urine when worn inside a person's underwear.

Per- and Polyfluoroalkyl Substances (PFAS)- They are a combination of more than eight thousand man made chemicals that possess an undetermined shelf life.

Petrol- Derived from petroleum, in liquid form it becomes fuel for most motor vehicles.

Petroleum- Common names are oil, crude, or petrol, it is a substance that occurs in certain places without any external assistance in the form of a hydrocarbon.

Plymouth Belvedere (1968)- A 1960's era four door sedan with a (318 v8) engine.

Pokey- Used as an informal adjective to describe a dreary location or facility that may be overcrowded with people in unfavorable environments.

Police Academy- Training facilities where Law Enforcement Agencies send their recruits to receive specialized training and certification to become enforcement officers.

Police / Sheriff / Law Enforcement- In general terms, their role is to protect life, property, investigate reports of crime, and keep the peace. In other respects, their primary functions are somewhat different. The Sheriff, for example, is an elected official who is responsible for the administration of the County Jail, and whose jurisdiction also encompasses the unincorporated areas of a County. Most Police Departments jurisdictions are usually contained within their municipalities.

Polish Journal of Environmental Studies- An organization that releases extremely important written documents on relevant topics that involve different types of harmful toxins or contaminants found in the air, dirt, refuse, and other organic matter. It may also invent or discover new procedures and tools for studying or determining ways of preventing or minimizing the advent of contaminants to name a few of its mandates.

Polycyclic Aromatic Hydrocarbons (PAH's)- They are a category of natural compounds that form into several aromatic circular objects when substances such as wood or oil are burned.

Potable Water- Water that is pure and is useful for drinking or cooking.

Potency- The ability of a physically developed male to attain and maintain an erection for the period it may take to reach orgasm.

Prisoner(s)- A person or persons held in confined quarters pending the outcome of a court hearing or upon conviction of a crime.

Prostate Biopsy- A medical procedure performed in a urologist's office using specific instruments that contain needles used to extract tissue samples from the prostate.

Prostate Cancer- Cancer or disease that has formed or developed in the body. Prostate Cancer Surgery- An operation or surgical procedure performed by a surgeon who will remove the prostate gland.

Prostate Gland- An organ in the body often attributed to the male sex.

Prostate Specific Antigen (PSA)- A test of a male subject's blood usually to determine whether cancer may be present.

Prostatitis- Disruption or discomfort of the prostate in some instances as a result of inflammation.

Radiation- It is the production or conveyance of energy in the form of waves or minute portions of matter.

Recovery Room- A secondary aftercare area in a hospital or other surgical facility where patients are monitored after undergoing an operation or medical procedure.

Refuse- Usually in solid form, it is trash or garbage that is gathered, collected, and transported to a dump site for processing.

Researcher- A student or professional who gathers, compiles, and presents information in a specific field of study.

Reusable Underwear- Underwear designed for men or women equipped with special material that absorbs bladder leaks. The underwear may be washed and reused repeatedly.

Robotic Surgery- An operation or medical procedure often performed by a trained surgeon who manipulates artificial arms while handling surgical instruments during surgery.

Ro.co/ Sparks- An online source for men who may seek consultation and treatment from a provider for erectile dysfunction.

Savings and Loan- A financial institution that accepts deposits into customers accounts and often uses those funds to offer and make mortgage loans to home buyers.

Self-Management- The practice of handling one's own personal matters, care, or needs.

Sexual Function- Refers to how a person's body may behave or respond during various phases of sexual activity.

Side Effects- A potential result or unfavorable effect from a specific medication or treatment.

Special Protective Apparel- Specific clothing or equipment designed to help protect the wearer from certain harmful environments or circum- stances.

Spinal Epidural- The administration of specific medication into a certain area of a person's body to relieve the sensation of pain for a certain period using a needle.

Surgeon- A medical professional who usually has been trained and board certified to perform surgical procedures.

Surgery- An area of care in health or medicine that provides or offers possible solutions for many illnesses or injuries with operations.

Surgical Intervention- The act or process of performing surgery on a subject to address, explore, or diagnose a condition.

Suspect- An individual or individuals believed to have committed a crime or to have violated a law.

Technician (Phlebotomist)- A person trained or certified to draw blood for examination or other purpose by piercing a subject's vein or fingers.

Toxin(s)- A type of foreign substance derived from a plant or animal that may produce microscopic living organisms capable of causing disease in a person's body.

Turnout Gear- Personal protective equipment worn by firefighters. Usually, a specifically treated or designed coat, pant, or footwear used to prevent or protect the wearer from injury to the body.

Ultrasound- Emission or vibrations transmitted by ultrasonic frequencies to produce a picture of a person's internal organs.

Uniform- Identical clothing or material of specific color, pattern, or markings worn by the same persons or members of an organization or facility.

Urinary Collection Bag- A device worn by a person designed to capture, hold, and dispense urine.

Urinary Incontinence- The inability to control or prevent the involuntary leakage of urine without the aid of some form of intervention.

Urologist- A medical professional who has been trained to treat men or women who may experience dysfunction within the urinary system.

Viagra®- A type of medication that may be prescribed for the treatment of male erectile dysfunction.

Virth Incontinence Clamp- A penile device developed for men who may suffer from urinary incontinence.

Wear-ever® Incontinence Underwear for Men- A brand of reusable underwear designed for men and women who may suffer from urinary incontinence or urine leakage.

EDITORIAL CONTRIBUTOR(s)
Dr. Shahrad Aynehchi, MD, FACS

Connect with Taryton on Social Media:

Instagram @simp.lelist4u
hopesanddreams1932@outlook.com